ANTIBIOTICS

THINGS YOU SHOULD KNOW
(QUESTIONS AND ANSWERS)

By Rumi Michael Leigh

Introduction

I would like to thank and congratulate you for purchasing this book, " *Antibiotics, things you should know (questions and answers)*" series.

This book will help you understand, revise and have a good general knowledge and keywords of Antibiotics.

Thanks again for purchasing this book, I hope you enjoy it!

Chapter 1

1) What are antibiotics ?

- Antibiotics are substances that fight bacterial infections.

2) Are all bacteria harmful ?

- No, not all bacteria are harmful. There are good and bad bacteria.

3) What is a microbiome ?

- A microbiome is a bacterium that lives in our body.

4) Do antibiotics only affect the bad bacteria ?

- No, antibiotics can also affect the good bacteria.

5) Do antibiotics act on viruses ?

- No, antibiotics don't act on viruses.

6) Why do antibiotics not act on viruses ?

- Antibiotics do not act on viruses because viruses have a different structure than the structure of bacteria.

7) What are the forms of antibiotics ?

-   Antibiotics can be in a pill form or in an intravenous fluid form.

8) Do bacteria have a cell wall ?

-   Yes, bacteria have a cell wall.

9) What are anaerobes bacteria ?

-   Anaerobes are bacteria that can thrive in the absence of oxygen.

10) Where are anaerobes bacteria mostly found in the body ?

-   Anaerobes bacteria are mostly found in the gastro intestinal tract.

Chapter 2

1) What is the cell wall made up of ?

- The cell wall is made up of polysaccharides and pentapeptide.

2) Do human cells have a cell wall ?

- No, human cells do not have a cell wall.

3) Is a cell membrane the same as a cell wall ?

- No, a cell membrane is not the same as a cell wall.

4) What is the main difference between a cell membrane and a cell wall ?

- The main difference between a cell membrane and a cell wall is that all types of cells have cell membranes but a cell wall is only present in plants, fungi, algae, and bacteria.

5) Give an example of an antibiotic that attacks the cell membrane of a bacteria.

- Polymyxin is an example of an antibiotic that attacks the cell membrane of a bacteria.

6) Give an example of an antibiotic that attacks the cell wall of a bacteria.

- Penicillin is an example of an antibiotic that attacks the cell wall of a bacteria.

7) What does Penicillin treat ?

- Penicillin treats syphilis, streptococcal, etc.

8) What is an enzyme ?

- An enzyme is a protein molecule that accelerates a chemical reaction.

9) What is a nosocomial infection ?

- A nosocomial infection is an infection contracted from a care setting (hospital, clinic, etc.)

10) What is pharmacokinetics ?

- Pharmacokinetics describes how drugs move and is used in the body.

Chapter 3

1) What is a targeted antibiotic ?

- A targeted antibiotic is an antibiotic that attacks a particular kind of bacteria.

2) When is a targeted antibiotic usually prescribed ?

- A targeted antibiotic is usually prescribed when the bacteria causing the infection is known.

3) What is a broad-spectrum antibiotic ?

- A broad-spectrum antibiotic is an antibiotic that attacks different kinds of bacteria.

4) When is a broad-spectrum antibiotic usually prescribed ?

- A broad-spectrum antibiotic is usually prescribed when the bacteria causing the infection is unknown.

5) What are the two main actions of an antibiotic ?

- The two main actions of an antibiotic are its bacteriostatic and bactericidal actions.

6) Do bacteriostatic antibiotics kill bacteria ?

- No, bacteriostatic antibiotics do not kill bacteria.

7) What is a bacteriostatic action of an antibiotic ?

- A bacteriostatic action of an antibiotic is an action that inhibits the multiplication of bacteria.

8) What is a bactericidal action of an antibiotic ?

- A bactericidal action of an antibiotic is an action that destroys/kills bacteria.

9) Can an antibiotic have both bacteriostatic and bactericidal actions ?

- Yes, an antibiotic can have both bacteriostatic and bactericidal actions.

10) What form is an antibiotic in an infected site ?

- An antibiotic is in an active form in an infected site.

Chapter 4

1) What is a coagulase ?

- A coagulase is a protein enzyme produced by microorganisms such as certain bacteria that convert fibrinogen to fibrin.

2) What is fibrinogen ?

- Fibrinogen is a protein that takes part in blood clotting.

3) What is fibrin ?

- Fibrin is a protein produced by fibrinogen that takes part in blood clotting.

4) Where can bacteria be found ?

- Bacteria can be found almost everywhere in our surrounding, even within us.

5) Can two antibiotics be combined and used on a patient ?

- Yes, two antibiotics can be used on a patient.

6) What is the benefit of combining two antibiotics ?

- The benefit of combining two antibiotics is to obtain better efficacy.

7) What is a symbiotic relationship between a bacterium and its host ?

- A symbiotic relationship between a bacterium and its host is a beneficial relationship between the bacterium and its host.

8) Can some types of antibiotics stop growth in adolescents ?

- Yes, some types of antibiotics can stop growth in adolescents.

9) How do some types of antibiotics stop growth in adolescents ?

- Some types of antibiotics can stop growth in adolescents by interfering with the epiphyseal cartilage.

10) What are prophylactics ?

- Prophylactics are medicines used to prevent disease.

Chapter 5

1) What is the shape of a coccus bacterium ?

- A coccus bacterium has a spherical shape.

2) What is the shape of a bacilli bacterium ?

- A bacilli bacterium has a rod shape.

3) Do Gram positive bacteria have an outer cell membrane ?

- No, Gram positive bacteria do not have an outer cell membrane.

4) Do Gram negative bacteria have an outer cell membrane ?

- Yes, Gram negative bacteria have an outer cell membrane.

5) What is pseudomonas ?

- Pseudomonas is Gram-negative bacteria.

6) Do all pseudomonas cause infections?

- No, not all pseudomonas cause infections.

7) What are atypical bacteria ?

- Atypical bacteria are bacteria with unusual cellular structures.

8) What is the color of an atypical bacteria with gram staining ?

- Atypical bacteria have no color with gram staining.

9) Are atypical bacteria gram positive ?

- No, atypical bacteria are not gram positive.

10) Are atypical bacteria gram negative ?

- No, atypical bacteria are not gram negative.

Chapter 6

1) What is the staining of a Gram-positive bacterium?

- The staining of a Gram-positive bacterium is violet.

2) What is the staining of a Gram-negative bacterium ?

- The staining of a Gram-negative bacterium is pink.

3) How is the wall of a Gram-positive bacterium ?

- Gram-positive bacterium has a thick wall.

4) How is the structure of a Gram-positive bacterium?

- Gram-positive bacterium has a simple structure.

5) How is the wall of a Gram-negative bacterium ?

- Gram-negative bacterium has a lesser thicker wall than that of a Gram-positive bacterium.

6) How is the structure of a Gram-negative bacterium ?

- The structure of a Gram-negative bacterium is complex.

7) How do antibiotics inhibit bacterial wall synthesis?

- Antibiotics inhibit bacterial wall synthesis by blocking the assembly of protein and lipid components.

8) How do antibiotics inhibit the synthesis of the cytoplasmic membrane ?

- Antibiotics inhibit the synthesis of the cytoplasmic membrane by entering the cell and altering the structure of the cytoplasmic membrane.

9) How do antibiotics inhibit the protein synthesis of bacteria ?

- Antibiotics inhibit the protein synthesis of bacteria by bridging the DNA filaments.

Chapter 7

1) What is neutropenia ?

- Neutropenia is a low level of neutrophils.

2) What are neutrophils ?

- Neutrophils are a type of white blood cells.

3) What is the function of neutrophils ?

- Neutrophils combat infections.

4) What is leucopenia ?

- Leucopenia is a reduction of the number of leukocytes.

5) What is Quincke's Edema ?

- Quincke's Edema is a frequent swelling of the deeper layer of the skin or mucosa.

6) What is another name for Quincke's Edema ?

- Another name for Quincke's Edema is Angioneurotic edema.

7) What is anuria ?

- Anuria is when the kidney can no longer produce urine.

8) What is oliguria ?

- Oliguria is a low urine output.

9) What is endocarditis ?

- Endocarditis is an inflammation of the endocardium due to an infection.

10) What is urticaria ?

- Urticaria, also known as hives is a skin inflammation that produces rash due to an allergic reaction.

Chapter 8

1) What is thrombocytopenia ?

- Thrombocytopenia is a low level of thrombocytes.

2) What is another name for thrombocytes ?

- Another name for thrombocytes is platelets.

3) What is the function of thrombocytes ?

- Thrombocytes aid in blood clotting.

4) What is pruritus ?

- Pruritus is itching of the skin.

5) What is candidiasis ?

- Candidiasis is a fungal infection caused by Candida.

6) What is hemolytic anemia ?

- Hemolytic anemia is a disorder in which there is rapid destruction of erythrocytes.

7) What is an anaphylactic shock ?

- An anaphylactic shock is a severe allergic reaction that causes the body to be over sensitive.

8) What is Salmonella ?

- Salmonella is a common bacterial disease that causes infection in the gastrointestinal tract.

9) What are the common causes of Salmonella ?

- The common causes of Salmonella are water and food contamination.

10) What is Klebsiella ?

- Klebsiella is a Gram-negative bacterial infection.

Chapter 9

1) What is the minimum inhibitory concentration of an antibiotic ?

- The minimum inhibitory concentration of an antibiotic is the lowest concentration of an antibiotic capable of inhibiting the multiplication of bacteria after 18 to 24 hours of contact at 37 degrees.

2) What is the minimum inhibitory concentration of an antibiotic ?

- The minimum inhibitory concentration of an antibiotic is the lowest concentration of an antibiotic that allows it to destroy 99.9% of bacteria after 18 to 24 hours of contact.

3) What is the route of administration of antibiotics for serious infections ?

- For serious infections, the route of administration of antibiotics is the parenteral route.

4) What is a parenteral administration ?

- A parenteral administration is the administration of a medicine on other parts of the body except the alimentary tract.

5) What are the routes of eliminating antibiotics ?

-   The routes of eliminating antibiotics are the urinary and the hepatic routes.

6) What is the normal flora of urine ?

-   Urine has no normal flora.

7) What is the normal flora of the blood ?

-   Blood has no normal flora.

Chapter 10

1) What are the allergic reactions caused by the side effects of antibiotics ?

- Allergic reactions caused by the side effects of antibiotics are rash, Quincke's edema, urticaria, pruritus, anaphylactic shock, etc.

2) Is an anaphylactic shock a life-threatening condition ?

- Yes, an anaphylactic shock could be a life-threatening condition.

3) What are the side effects of antibiotics ?

- The side effects of antibiotics are hypotension, ototoxicity, muscle pain, joint pain, allergic reactions, neurological disorders, digestive disorders, kidney disorders, nephrotoxicity, and hematological disorders.

4) What are the digestive disorders caused by the side effects of antibiotics ?

- Digestive disorders caused by the side effects of antibiotics are nausea, vomiting, candidiasis, diarrhea, abdominal pain, etc.

5) What are the hematological disorders caused by the side effects of antibiotics ?

- Hematological disorders caused by the side effects of antibiotics are hemolytic anemia, leukopenia, neutropenia, thrombocytopenia, etc.

6) What are the neurological disorders caused by the side effects of antibiotics ?

- Neurological disorders caused by the side effects of antibiotics are insomnia, headaches, drowsiness, etc.

7) What are the kidney disorders caused by the side effects of antibiotics ?

- Kidney disorders caused by the side effects of antibiotics include kidney stones, anuria, oliguria, etc.

8) What are the ototoxicity disorders caused by the side effects of antibiotics ?

- The ototoxicity disorders caused by the side effects of antibiotics are tinnitus, balance disorders, etc.

Chapter 11

1) What can Amoxicillin treat ?

- Amoxicillin can treat salmonella, meningitis, urinary tract infection, respiratory tract infection, etc.

2) What is Isoniazid ?

- Isoniazid is an antibiotic used for the treatment of tuberculosis.

3) What can cephalosporins treat ?

- Cephalosporins treat meningitis, pseudomonas, Klebsiella, etc.

4) What are Macrolides ?

- Macrolides are bacteriostatic antibiotics.

5) Give some examples of Macrolide antibiotics.

- Some examples of Macrolide antibiotics are Erythromycin, Clarithromycin, Fidaxomicin, and Zithromax.

6) What do Macrolides antibiotics treat ?

- Macrolides antibiotics treat gastro-intestinal infection, pneumonia, sexually transmitted diseases, Helicobacter Pylori, etc.

7) What is Pneumonia ?

-   Pneumonia is an infection that causes the inflammation of the air sac of the lungs.

8) What are Helicobacter Pylori ?

-   Helicobacter Pylori is a bacterial infection in the digestive tract that causes complications such as sores, ulcers, that can eventually lead to stomach cancer.

9) Is Helicobacter Pylori Gram positive or Gram-negative bacteria ?

-   Helicobacter Pylori are Gram-negative bacteria.

Chapter 12

1) What are Amino-Glycosides ?

- Amino-Glycosides are bactericidal antibiotics.

2) Give examples of Amino-Glycoside antibiotics.

- Some examples of Amino-Glycoside antibiotics are Plazomicin, Gentamicin, Amikacin, Tobramycin, etc.

3) What do Amino-Glycosides treat ?

- Amino Glycosides treat pneumonia, meningitis, urinary tract infection, etc.

4) What does Rifampicin treat ?

- Rifampicin treats leprosy, tuberculosis, legionnaires' disease, etc.

5) What is legionnaires' disease ?

- Legionnaires disease is a serious form of pneumonia caused by legionella bacteria.

6) What is the action of Rifampicin ?

- Rifampicin inhibits the DNA dependent RNA polymerase enzyme.

7) What is the function of RNA polymerase ?

- RNA polymerase is used for the transcription of DNA to mRNA.

8) What is the action of Daptomycin antibiotics ?

- Daptomycin antibiotics inhibit the synthesis of DNA and RNA.

9) What are tetracycline antibiotics ?

- Tetracycline antibiotics are bacteriostatic antibiotics.

10) What do tetracycline antibiotics treat ?

- Tetracycline antibiotics treat urinary tract infection, respiratory tract infection, malaria, acne, Lyme disease, anthrax, pneumonia, etc.

Chapter 13

1) Give an example of an antibiotic that inhibits the metabolization of folic acid in bacteria.

- Sulfonamide is an antibiotic that inhibits the metabolization of folic acid in bacteria.

2) Give an example of an antibiotic that inhibits the synthesis of DNA in bacteria.

- Rifamycin is an antibiotic that inhibits the synthesis of DNA in bacteria.

3) Give an example of an antibiotic that inhibits the synthesis of proteins in bacteria.

- Streptomycin is an antibiotic that inhibits the synthesis of proteins in bacteria.

Conclusion

Thank you again for purchasing this book. I hope it has helped you in your journey to understanding Antibiotics.

Thank you.